NOURISH & FIT

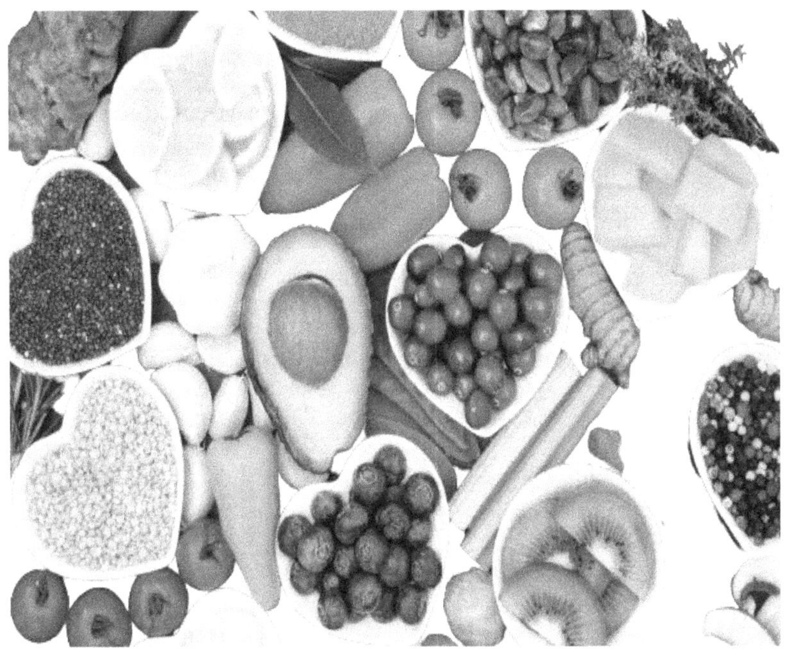

Quick and Easy Weight Loss Recipes With Wholesome 30-Day Meal Plan

FELICIA WINDROW

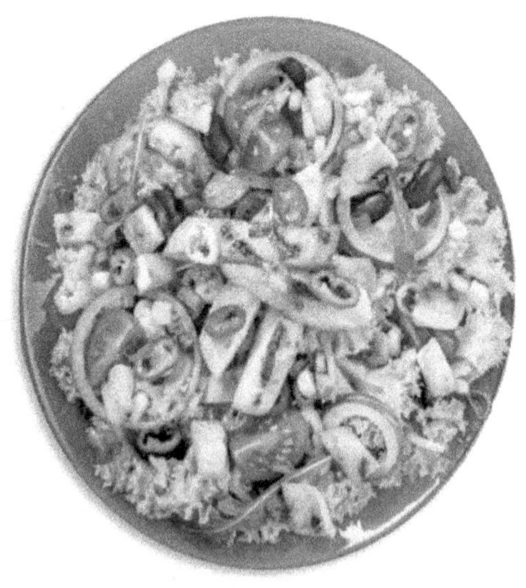

TABLE OF CONTENT

INTRODUCTION

Patricia has been struggling with her weight for years and has tried different diet and exercise programs, but nothing seemed to work.

Patricia was feeling frustrated and hopeless until she came across the book titled 'Nourish and Fit' which she got for a few dollars. This book has completely changed her life after following instructions in it.

This book titled 'Nourish and Fit' is an amazing resource that provides a comprehensive approach to health and fitness. It is filled with practical advice and tips on how to make healthy lifestyle changes that will help you reach your fitness goals.

This book is easy to understand and provides detailed information on nutrition, exercise, and lifestyle changes.

The book has helped Patricia to make healthier food choices and to create a balanced diet that is tailored to her individual needs by not procrastinating on its basics. She has also been able to incorporate regular exercise into her daily routine, which has helped her to lose weight and gain muscle.

This book has also helped Patricia to develop a positive attitude towards her body and to appreciate her body for what it is. She has learned to be kind to herself and to focus on the positive aspects of her body.

This book has been a valuable resource in her journey to health and fitness. It has helped her to make positive changes to her lifestyle and towards reaching her fitness goals.

I would highly recommend this book to anyone who is looking to make healthy lifestyle changes and to reach their fitness goals in a short period with ease.

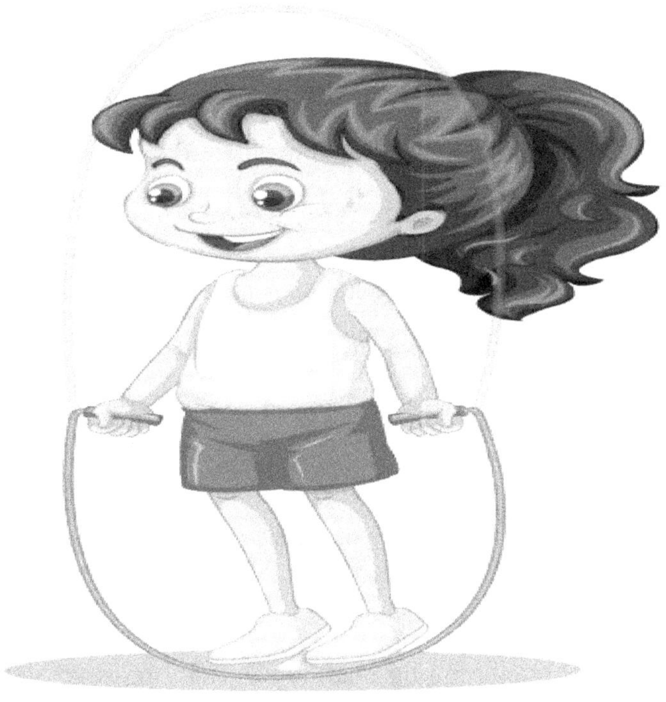

CHAPTER 1

The Importance of Healthy Eating

1. Improved Mood: Eating healthy can help improve your mood and reduce stress.

Eating a balanced diet can help you feel more energized and alert, and can help you stay focused and productive.

2. Weight Management: Eating healthy can help you maintain a healthy weight.

Eating a balanced diet that includes plenty of fruits, vegetables, and whole grains can help you maintain a healthy weight and reduce your risk of obesity.

3. Reduced Risk of Disease: Eating healthy can help reduce your risk of developing chronic diseases such as heart disease, diabetes, and cancer.

Eating a balanced diet that includes plenty of fruits, vegetables, and whole grains can help reduce your risk of developing these diseases.

4. Improved Energy Levels: Eating healthy can help improve your energy levels.

Eating a balanced diet that includes plenty of fruits, vegetables, and whole grains can help you feel more energized and alert.

5. Improved Digestion: Eating healthy can help improve your digestion.

Eating a balanced diet that includes plenty of fruits, vegetables, and whole grains can help your body break down and absorb nutrients more efficiently.

6. Improved Immune System: Eating healthy can help improve your immune system.

Eating a balanced diet that includes plenty of fruits, vegetables, and whole grains can help your body fight off infections and illnesses.

7. Improved Cognitive Function: Eating healthy can help improve your cognitive function.

Eating a balanced diet that includes plenty of fruits, vegetables, and whole grains can help your brain function better and can help you stay focused and productive.

8. Reduced Risk of Osteoporosis: Eating healthy can help reduce your risk of dev osteoporosis.

Eating a balanced diet that has plenty of calcium-rich foods can help strengthen your bones and reduce your risk of high osteoporosis.

9. Reduced Risk of Depression: Eating healthy can help reduce your risk of developing depression.

Eating a balanced diet that includes plenty of fruits, vegetables, and whole grains can help improve your mood and reduce your risk of developing depression. 10. Improved Skin Health: Eating healthy can help improve your skin health.

Eating a balanced diet that includes plenty of fruits, vegetables, and whole grains can help keep your skin looking healthy and can help reduce your risk of developing skin problems.

11. Reduced Risk of Heart Disease: Eating healthy can help reduce your risk of developing heart disease.

Eating a balanced diet that includes plenty of fruits, vegetables, and whole grains can help reduce your risk of developing heart disease.

12. Improved Sleep Quality: Eating healthy can help improve your sleep quality.

Eating a balanced diet that includes plenty of fruits, vegetables, and whole grains can help you get a better night's sleep and can help you wake up feeling more refreshed.

13. Reduced Risk of Type 2 Diabetes: Eating healthy can help reduce your risk of developing type 2 diabetes.

Eating a balanced diet that includes plenty of fruits, vegetables, and whole grains can help reduce your risk of developing type 2 diabetes.

14. Improved Bone Health: Eating healthy can help improve your bone health.

Eating a balanced diet that includes plenty of calcium-rich foods can help strengthen your bones and reduce your risk of developing osteoporosis.

15. Reduced Risk of Cancer: Eating healthy can help reduce your risk of developing cancer.

Eating a balanced diet that includes plenty of fruits, vegetables, and whole grains can help reduce your risk of developing cancer.

16. Improved Mental Health: Eating healthy can help improve your mental health.

Eating a balanced diet that includes plenty of fruits, vegetables, and whole grains can help improve your mood and reduce your risk of developing depression.

17. Improved Physical Performance: Eating healthy can help improve your physical performance.

Eating a balanced diet that includes plenty of fruits, vegetables, and whole grains can help you stay energized and can help you perform better during physical activities.

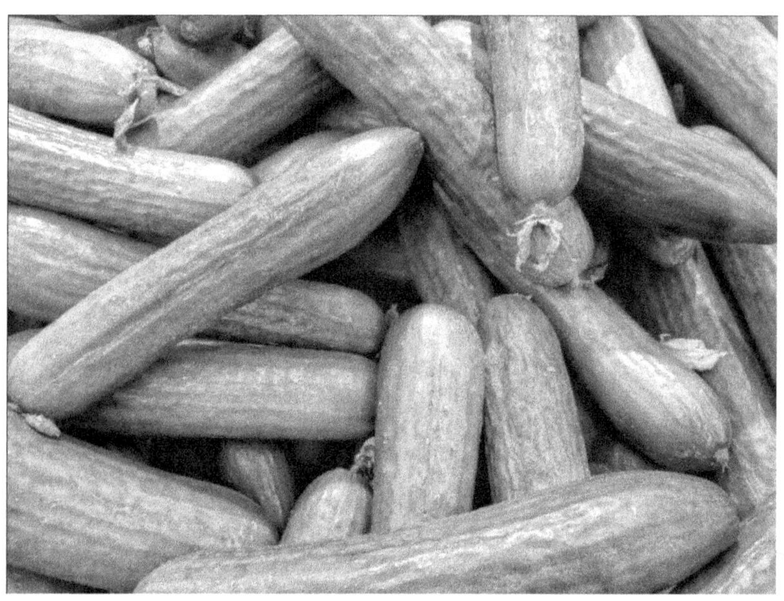

18. Reduced Risk of High Blood Pressure: Eating healthy can help reduce your risk of developing high blood pressure.

Eating a balanced diet that includes plenty of fruits, vegetables, and whole grains can help reduce your risk of developing high blood pressure.

19. Improved Vision: Eating healthy can help improve your vision.

Eating a balanced diet that includes plenty of fruits, vegetables, and whole grains can help improve your vision and can help reduce your risk of developing vision problems.

20. Improved Overall Health: Eating healthy can help improve your overall health.

Eating a balanced diet that includes plenty of fruits, vegetables, and whole grains can help you feel better and can help you stay healthy.

Benefits of Quick and Easy Recipes

1. Saves time and effort in meal preparation.

2. Ideal for busy individuals with limited time for cooking.

3. Provides a convenient option for those whose always on the go.

4. Reduces stress associated with complicated recipes and extensive cooking processes.

5. Allows for more time to focus on other activities or responsibilities.

6. Can be prepared and enjoyed by novice cooks without extensive culinary skills.

7. Offers a wide range of options for quick and nutritious meals.

8. Helps maintain a balanced diet by providing quick access to healthy ingredients.

9. Encourages experimentation with different flavors and ingredients.

10. Minimizes excessive consumption of processed or unhealthy fast food options.

11. Provides opportunities for creative and customizable dishes.

12. Promotes portion control and mindful eating.

13. Reduces food waste as quick and easy recipes often utilize pantry staples.

14. Enables preparation of meals in advance for easy reheating or meal planning.

15. Enhances productivity by allowing individuals to spend less time in the kitchen.

16. Suitable for individuals with dietary restrictions, as it is simple to make ingredients.

17. Inspires confidence and enjoyment in cooking for those who may otherwise find it challenging or intimidating.

18. Economical approach to cooking, as it requires fewer ingredients and utensils.

19. It can be an option for individuals on a tight budget.

20. Encourages family bonding and shared meal experiences, as quick and easy recipes can be organized and enjoyed together.

How to Set Realistic Weight Loss Goals?

Setting realistic weight loss goals that prioritize nourishing and keeping your body fit is essential for long-term success. Here are specific ways to help you achieve these goals:

1. Consult a Healthcare Professional: Before starting a weight loss journey, consult a doctor or a registered dietitian. They are able to evaluate your present health and make tailored recommendations.

2. Set Specific Goals: Clearly define your weight loss goals in terms of pounds or inches, but also consider non-scale goals like improved energy, better sleep, or enhanced mood.

3. Create a Realistic Timeline: Don't rush your weight loss. Aim for a gradual, sustainable rate of about 1-2 pounds per week. Rapid weight loss can be dangerous to maintain.

4. Focus on Nutrition: Emphasize a balanced diet like plenty of fruits, vegetables, lean proteins, whole grains, and healthy fats. Steer clear of severe diets like eliminating entire food groupings.

5. Portion Control: Learn to portion your meals appropriately. To help regulate portion sizes and minimize overeating, use smaller plates.

6. Regular Exercise: Combine a balanced diet with regular physical activity. Aim for at least 150 minutes of moderate-intensity aerobic exercise often, alongside strength training for muscle maintenance.

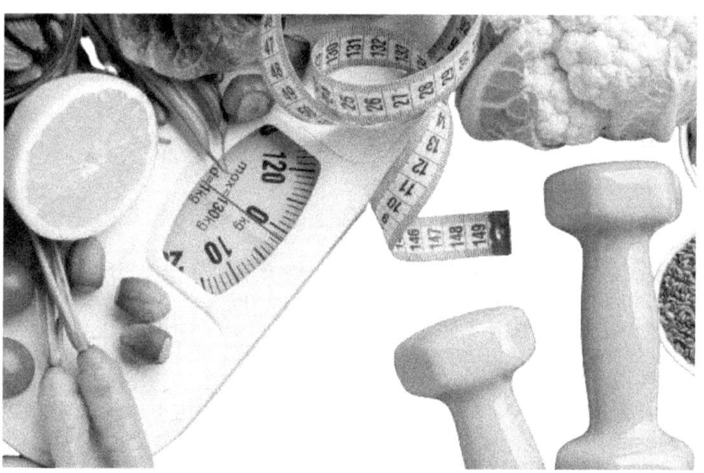

7. Hydration: To keep hydrated, drink lots of water. Sometimes, thirst is mistaken for hunger. Your appetite can be moderate by drinking water.

8. Track Your Progress: Keep a journal or use a fitness app to record your meals, exercise, and feelings. You can use this to spot trends and potential improvement areas.

9. Set Realistic Expectations: Understand that weight loss plateaus and fluctuations are normal. Don't be discouraged by minor setbacks. Focus on the bigger picture and your overall health.

10. Seek Support: Share your goals with friends or family who can provide encouragement and accountability. Join a support group for those trying to lose weight, or work with a nutritionist or personal trainer.

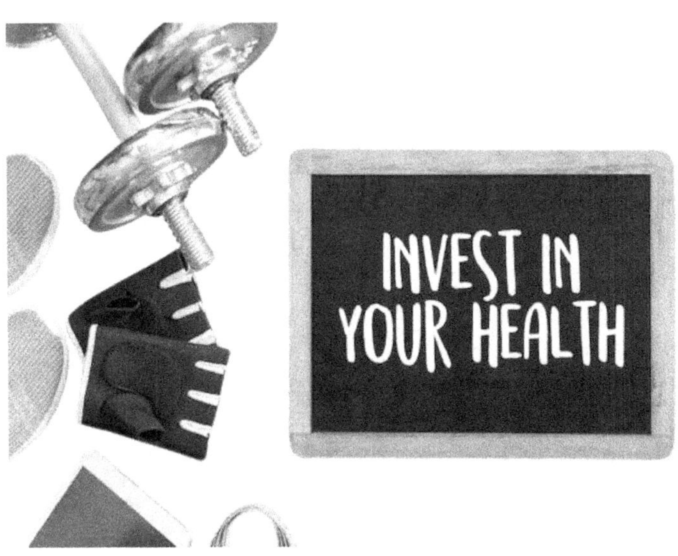

CHAPTER 2

Understanding Weight Loss

Weight loss is a complex process that involves understanding the body's metabolism, hormones, and lifestyle choices. It is important to understand the basics of weight loss in order to achieve and maintain a healthy weight.

The most important factor in weight loss is creating a calorie deficit, which means burning more calories than you consume.

This can be done through diet and exercise. Eating a balanced diet with plenty of fruits, vegetables, and lean proteins can help to reduce calorie intake.

Exercise is also important for weight loss, as it helps to burn calories and builds muscle. Whereas, understanding the body's hormones and metabolism can help to regulate weight loss.

Hormones such as insulin, leptin, and ghrelin can affect hunger and satiety, and understanding how these hormones work can help to regulate weight loss. Also lifestyle choices such as sleep, stress, and alcohol consumption can also affect weight loss.

Understanding the basics of weight loss can help to create a successful plan for achieving and maintaining a healthy weight.

The Science behind Weight Loss

Weight loss is a common goal for many people, whether it be for health reasons or to improve physical appearance. While it may seem straightforward, there is actually a science behind weight loss that involves understanding the body's metabolism, energy balance, and the role of nutrition and exercise.

To understand weight loss, it is important to grasp the concept of energy balance. Our body requires energy to perform various functions such as breathing, digestion, and physical activity. This energy is obtained from the calories we consume through food and beverages.

When the number of calories consumed equals the number of calories burned, it results in weight maintenance. However, when the calories consumed are greater than the calories burned, excess energy is stored in the form of fat, leading to weight gain. On the other hand, when the calories burned exceed the calories consumed, this creates a calorie deficit, resulting in weight loss.

One pound of body weight is roughly equivalent to 3,500 calories. Therefore, to lose one pound, a calorie deficit of 3,500 calories needs to be created.

This can be achieved through a combination of reducing calorie intake and increasing physical activity. However, it is important to note that weight loss should be achieved in a healthy and sustainable manner. Rapid weight loss methods often result in muscle loss and nutrient deficiencies, and can be detrimental to overall health.

Nutrition plays a crucial role in weight loss. Consuming a balanced diet that is rich in fruits, vegetables, lean proteins, whole grains, and healthy fats helps provide essential nutrients while keeping calorie intake in check.

A diet high in fiber and protein can help promote satiety and control hunger, making it easier to create a calorie deficit.

Exercise is another important component of weight loss. Regular physical activity helps increase energy expenditure, contributing to the calorie deficit needed for weight loss.

It also helps build lean muscle mass, which can boost metabolism and enhance fat burning. Combining cardiovascular exercises, such as revising or cycling with strength training exercises can yield optimal results.

It is important to understand that weight loss is not a linear process. It involves various factors such as genetics, hormones, sleep, stress, and overall lifestyle. It is normal to experience fluctuations in weight, and sustainable weight loss occurs gradually over time.

Weight loss is a complex process that involves understanding energy balance, nutrition, and exercise. It requires creating a calorie deficit through a combination of reducing calorie intake and increasing physical activity. It is important to approach weight loss in a healthy and sustainable manner.

Consulting with healthcare professionals, similar to registered dietitians or particular coaches, can give substantiated guidance and support throughout the weight loss trip. With the right knowledge and strategies, achieving and maintaining a healthy weight is attainable.

Factors Affecting Weight Loss

1. Diet: Eating a healthy, balanced diet that is low in calories and high in nutrients is essential for weight loss. Eating a diet high in reused foods, sugar, and unhealthy fats can lead to weight gain.

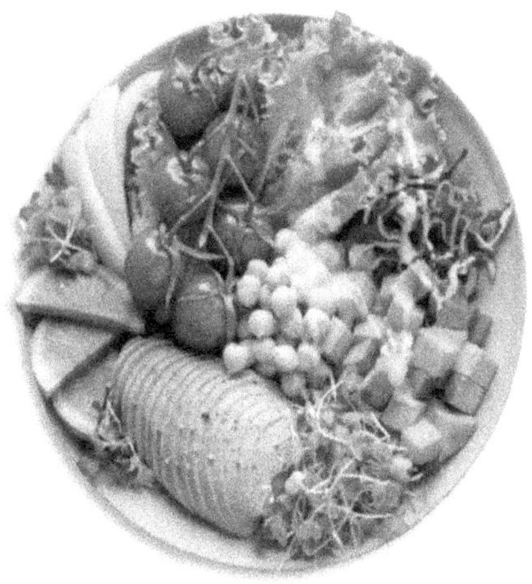

2. Exercise: Regular physical actions for weight loss are not necessitated. Exercise helps to burn calories and builds muscle, which can help to boost metabolism and burn more calories.

3. Stress: Stress can lead to overeating and weight gain. Finding ways to manage stress can help to reduce the risk of weight gain.

4. Sleep: Getting enough sleep is necessary for weight loss. Increased hunger and cravings brought on by a lack of sleep might result in overeating and weight gain.

5. Genetics: Genetics might affect how well you lose weight. It's possible that some people are genetically predisposed to acquiring or losing weight.

6. Medications: Certain medications can cause weight gain or make it harder to lose weight.

7. Hormones: Hormones can affect weight loss. Changes in hormones can lead to changes in appetite and metabolism, which affects weight.

8. Age: As people age, their metabolism slows down, which make losing weight difficult.

9. Medical Conditions: Certain medical conditions can make it harder to lose weight. These include thyroid disorders, diabetes, and polycystic ovary syndrome.

10. Environment: The environment can affect weight loss. Eating out more often or living in an area with limited access to healthy food can make it harder to lose weight.

11. Social Support: A supportive social network can help weight loss. Having people to talk to and encourage you can make it easier to stay on track.

12. Mindset: Having a positive mindset can help with weight loss. Believing that you can achieve your goals can help to motivate you and keep you on track.

13. Portion Control: Eating smaller portions can help with weight loss. Eat more regularly and in little quantities to reduce hunger and cravings.

14. Hydration: Staying hydrated is necessary for weight loss. Getting lots of water might aid in lowering cravings and hunger.

15. Supplements: Taking certain supplements can help with weight loss. These include protein powders, green tea extract, and pro biotic.

Healthy Weight Loss vs Crash Diets

Healthy weight loss and crash diets are very different approaches to losing weight.

Healthy weight loss is a gradual process that calls for creating lifestyle changes such as eating a balanced diet and exercising regularly. It is compulsory to focus on making sustainable changes that is time maintaining.

Crash diets, on the other hand, are extreme diets that involve drastic changes in eating habits and often involve cutting out entire food groups. These diets are often unsustainable and can lead to health problems.

Healthy weight loss is the best approach for long-term success. It involves making little changes to your diet and lifestyle that is time maintaining.

Eating a balanced diet that includes a variety of fruits, vegetables, whole grains, lean proteins, and healthy fats is compulsory for maintaining a healthy weight. Regular physical activity is also important for weight loss and overall health.

It is not of importance to use crash diets to lose weight over the long run. These diets often cut out entire food groups and can lead to nutrient deficiencies. They are also not maintainable and can lead to weight gain once the diet is left out. Crash diets can also lead to health problems such as fatigue, dehydration, and electrolyte imbalances.

Healthy weight loss is the best approach for long-term success. It involves making sustainable changes to your diet and lifestyle that is been preserved over time.

Crash diets are not compulsory since they might beget health issues and do not have long-term results.

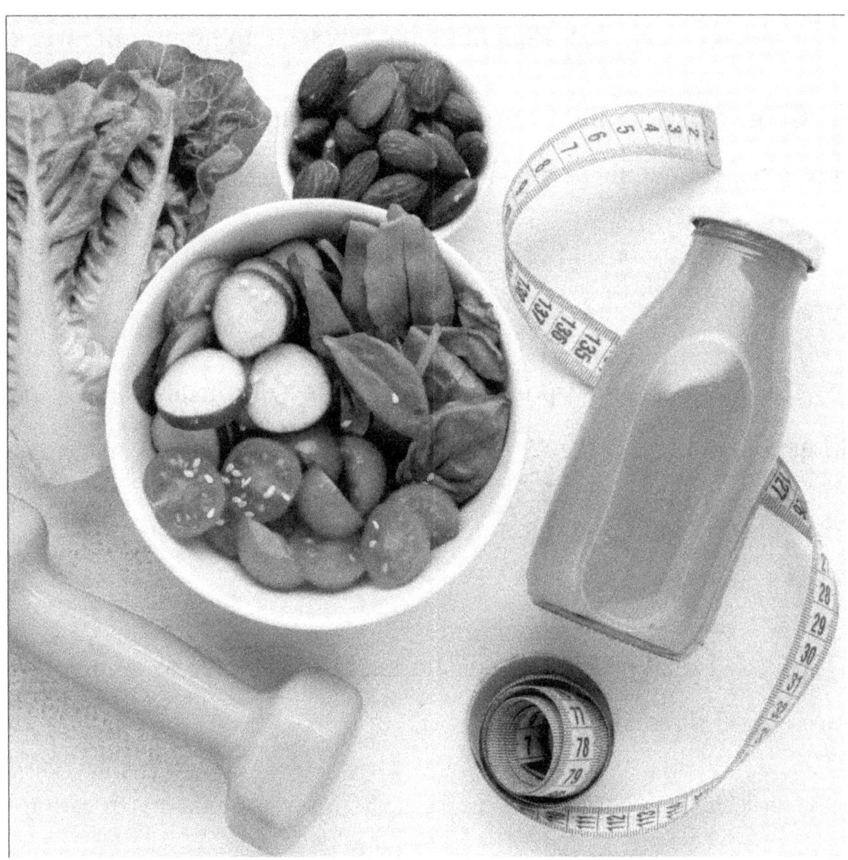

CHAPTER 3

Basics of Meal Plan

1. Set a budget: Decide how much you can afford to spend on groceries each week.

2. Make a grocery list: Plan out what you need to buy for the week.

3. Choose healthy foods: Focus on fresh fruits and vegetables, lean proteins, and whole grains.

4. Plan meals ahead of time: Decide what you'll make for breakfast, lunch, and dinner each day.

5. Use leftovers: Incorporate leftovers into your meal plan to save time and money.

6. Shop in bulk: Buy items like grains, beans, and nuts in bulk to save money.

7. Buy seasonal produce: Look for seasonal produce to get the best prices and flavors.

8. Cook in batches: Make extra servings of meals to freeze for later.

9. Store food properly: Store food in airtight containers to keep it fresh longer.

10. Eat mindfully: Enjoy your meals and be mindful of your portion sizes.

30-Day Weight-Loss Meal Plan

Day 1:

Breakfast: Oatmeal with banana and almond butter

Lunch: Grilled chicken salad with olive oil and lemon dressing

Snack: Greek yogurt with berries

Dinner: Baked salmon with roasted vegetables

Snack: Apple slices with peanut butter

Day 2:

Breakfast: Egg and vegetable scramble

Lunch: Quinoa and black bean burrito

Snack: Celery sticks with hummus

Dinner: Grilled chicken with roasted sweet potatoes

Snack: Air-popped popcorn

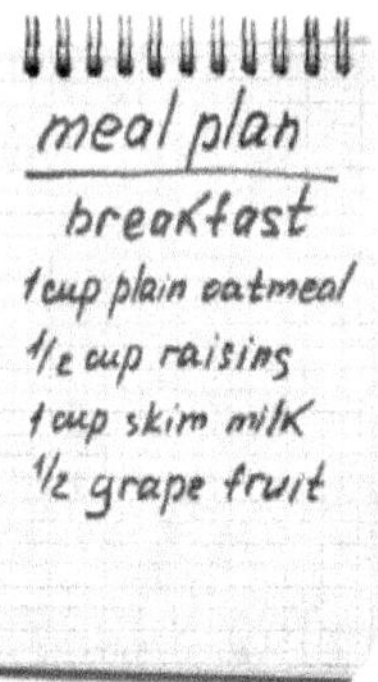

Day 3:

Breakfast: Avocado toast with poached egg

Lunch: Turkey wrap with lettuce, tomato, and avocado

Snack: Trail mix with nuts and dried fruit

Dinner: Baked cod with roasted asparagus

Snack: Greek yogurt with granola

Day 4:

Breakfast: Smoothie bowl with banana, berries, and almond milk

Lunch: Lentil soup with a side of whole-grain bread

Snack: Carrot sticks with hummus

Dinner: Grilled shrimp with quinoa and steamed vegetables

Snack: Apple slices with almond butter

Day 5:

Breakfast: Omelet with spinach, mushrooms, and feta cheese

Lunch: Tuna salad with celery and onion

Snack: Edamame

Dinner: Baked chicken with roasted Brussels sprouts

Snack: Popcorn with Parmesan cheese

Day 6:

Breakfast: Whole-grain toast with peanut butter and banana

Lunch: Rilled salmon with quinoa and steamed vegetables

Snack: Celery sticks with almond butter

Dinner: Baked cod with roasted potatoes

Snack: Greek yogurt with berries

Day 7:

Breakfast: Oatmeal with banana and walnuts

Lunch: Turkey wrap with lettuce, tomato, and avocado

Snack: Trail mix with nuts and dried fruit

Dinner: Grilled chicken with roasted sweet potatoes

Snack: Air-popped popcorn

Day 8:

Breakfast: Smoothie bowl with banana, berries, and almond milk

Lunch: Lentil soup with a side of whole-grain bread

Snack: Carrot sticks with hummus

Dinner: Baked cod with roasted asparagus

Snack: Greek yogurt with granola

Day 9:

Breakfast: Avocado toast with poached egg

Lunch: Quinoa and black bean burrito

Snack: Edamame

Dinner: Grilled shrimp with quinoa and steamed vegetables

Snack: Apple slices with almond butter

Day 10:

Breakfast: Egg and vegetable scramble

Lunch: Tuna salad with celery and onion

Snack: Celery sticks with hummus

Dinner: Baked chicken with roasted Brussels sprouts

Snack: Popcorn with Parmesan cheese

Day 11:

Breakfast: Whole-grain toast with peanut butter and banana

Lunch: Grilled salmon with quinoa and steamed vegetables

Snack: Apple slices with peanut butter

Dinner: Baked cod with roasted potatoes

Snack: Greek yogurt with berries

Day 12:

Breakfast: Omelet with spinach, mushrooms, and feta cheese

Lunch: Grilled chicken salad with olive oil and lemon dressing

Snack: Trail mix with nuts and dried fruit

Dinner: Grilled shrimp with quinoa and steamed vegetables

Snack: Air-popped popcorn

Day 13:

Breakfast: Smoothie bowl with banana, berries, and almond milk

Lunch: Lentil soup with a side of whole-grain bread

Snack: Celery sticks with almond butter

Dinner: Baked chicken with roasted Brussels sprouts

Snack: Greek yogurt with granola

Day 14:

Breakfast: Avocado toast with poached egg

Lunch: Quinoa and black bean burrito

Snack: Edamame

Dinner: Baked cod with roasted asparagus

Snack: Popcorn with Parmesan cheese

Day 15:

Breakfast: Oatmeal with banana and walnuts

Lunch: Turkey wrap with lettuce, tomato, and avocado

Snack: Carrot sticks with hummus

Dinner: Grilled salmon with quinoa and steamed vegetables

Snack: Apple slices with almond butter

Day 16:

Breakfast: Egg and vegetable scramble

Lunch: Tuna salad with celery and onion

Snack: Celery sticks with hummus

Dinner: Baked cod with roasted potatoes

Snack: Greek yogurt with berries

Day 16:

Breakfast: Whole-grain toast with peanut butter and banana

Lunch: Grilled chicken salad with olive oil and lemon dressing

Snack: Trail mix with nuts and dried fruit

Dinner: Grilled shrimp with quinoa and steamed vegetables

Snack: Air-popped popcorn

Day 17:

Breakfast: Smoothie bowl with banana, berries, and almond milk

Lunch: Lentil soup with a side of whole-grain bread

Snack: Carrot sticks with hummus

Dinner: Baked chicken with roasted Brussels sprouts

Snack: Greek yogurt with granola

Day 18:

Breakfast: Avocado toast with poached egg

Lunch: Quinoa and black bean burrito

Snack: Edamame

Dinner: Baked cod with roasted asparagus

Snack: Popcorn with Parmesan cheese

Day 19:

Breakfast: Omelet with spinach, mushrooms, and feta cheese

Lunch: Grilled salmon with quinoa and steamed vegetables

Snack: Apple slices with peanut butter

Dinner: Grilled shrimp with quinoa and steamed vegetables

Snack: Celery sticks with almond butter

Day 20:

Breakfast: Oatmeal with banana and walnuts

Lunch: Turkey wrap with lettuce, tomato, and avocado

Snack: Trail mix with nuts and dried fruit

Dinner: Baked chicken with roasted sweet potatoes

Snack: Air-popped popcorn

Day 21:

Breakfast: Smoothie bowl with banana, berries, and almond milk

Lunch: Lentil soup with a side of whole-grain bread

Snack: Carrot sticks with hummus

Dinner: Baked cod with roasted asparagus

Snack: Greek yogurt with granola

Day 22:

Breakfast: Avocado toast with poached egg

Lunch: Quinoa and black bean burrito

Snack: Edamame

Dinner: Grilled shrimp with quinoa and steamed vegetables

Snack: Apple slices with almond butter

Day 23:

Breakfast: Egg and vegetable scramble

Lunch: Tuna salad with celery and onion

Snack: Celery sticks with hummus

Dinner: Baked chicken with roasted Brussels sprouts

Snack: Popcorn with Parmesan cheese

Day 24:

Breakfast: Greek yogurt with fresh berries and a handful of almonds

Snack: Apple slices with almond butter

Lunch: Vegan Mediterranean lentil soup with a side salad

Snack: Carrots and hummus

Dinner: Curried sweet potato and peanut soup with a slice of whole-wheat baguette

Day 25:

Breakfast: Scrambled eggs with spinach and a slice of whole-grain toast

Snack: A small handful of mixed nuts

Lunch: Chicken and vegetable stir-fry with brown rice

Snack: Greek yogurt with honey and cinnamon

Dinner: Slow-cooker beef stew with a side salad

Day 26:

Breakfast: Overnight oats with chia seeds, almond milk, and fresh fruit

Snack: Baby carrots with ranch dressing

Lunch: Tomato and basil soup with a grilled cheese sandwich
Snack: A small apple with almond butter

Dinner: Baked salmon with roasted vegetables

Day 27:

Breakfast: Smoothie with spinach, banana, almond milk, and protein powder

Snack: Hard-boiled egg with a sprinkle of salt

Lunch: Chicken and vegetable soup with a side salad

Snack: Greek yogurt with fresh berries

Dinner: Slow-cooker chicken chili with a side of cornbread

Day 28:

Breakfast: Avocado toast with a fried egg

Snack: A small handful of trail mix

Lunch: Lentil and vegetable soup with a side salad

Snack: Sliced cucumber with hummus

Dinner: Slow-cooker vegetable stew with a side of garlic bread

Day 29:

Breakfast: Greek yogurt with granola and fresh fruit

Snack: A small apple with almond butter

Lunch: Turkey and vegetable soup with a side salad

Snack: Baby carrots with ranch dressing

Dinner: Slow-cooker beef and vegetable stew

Day 30:

Breakfast: Scrambled eggs with spinach and a slice of whole-grain toast

Snack: A small handful of mixed nuts

Lunch: Tomato and basil soup with a grilled cheese sandwich

Snack: Greek yogurt with honey and cinnamon

Dinner: Slow-cooker chicken and vegetable stew

Portion Control and Calorie Counting

Portion control and calorie counting are two of the most important aspects of weight loss. Portion management is a activity in controlling how much food you consume at one sitting. It helps to prevent overeating and can help you to reach your weight loss goals. Calorie counting is an endeavor of tracking the number of calories you consume each day. It helps to ensure that you are eating the right amount of calories to reach your weight loss goals.

Portion control can be achievable by using smaller plates and bowls, measuring out food, and avoiding second helpings. It is important to remember that portion sizes should be in your individual needs and goals.

Calorie counting can be by using a food diary or an app to track your daily intake. It is important to remember that calories are not the only factor in weight loss and that other factors such as exercise and nutrition are also important.

Portion control and calorie counting can be difficult to maintain, but with practice and dedication, they can be effective tool for weight loss. It is important to remember that weight loss is a journey and that it takes time and effort to reach your goals. Your weight loss objectives are attainable with the correct methods and commitment.

CHAPTER 4

Quick and Easy Recipes

Breakfast

1. Overnight Oats:

Ingredients:

Rolled oats, milk (or yogurt), honey, fruits, nuts.

Preparation:

In a jar, combine oats, milk/yogurt, and sweetener. Refrigerate overnight. Before serving, garnish with nuts and fruits.

Prep Time:

5 minutes (+ overnight refrigeration)

Nutritional Value:

High in fiber, protein, and antioxidants.

2. Avocado Toast:

Ingredients:

Bread, avocado, lemon juice, salt, pepper, red chili flakes, optional toppings (such as eggs, tomatoes, or feta cheese).

Preparation:

Toast the bread. Lemon juice, salt, and pepper used to mash avocado. Spread over toasted bread. Add toppings if desired.

Prep Time:

10 minutes

Nutritional Value:

Rich in vitamins, fiber, and good fats.

3. Vegetable Omelet:

Ingredients:

Eggs, vegetables (bell peppers, onions, mushrooms, spinach, etc.), salt, pepper, cheese (optional).

Preparation:

Beat eggs with salt and pepper. Sauté vegetables. Pour beaten eggs over vegetables. Cook until set. Add cheese if desired.

Prep Time:

15 minutes

Nutritional Value:

High in protein, vitamins, and minerals.

4. Greek Yogurt Parfait:

Ingredients:

Greek yogurt, granola, fruits, honey.

Preparation:

Layer Greek yogurt, granola, and fruits in a glass. Drizzle with honey.

Prep Time:

5 minutes

Nutritional Value:

Good source of protein, calcium, and fiber.

5. Peanut Butter Banana Smoothie:

Ingredients:

Banana, peanut butter, milk (or yogurt), honey, ice cubes.

Preparation:

Blend banana, peanut butter, milk/yogurt, honey, and ice cubes until smooth.

Prep Time:

5 minutes

Nutritional Value:

Provides protein, healthy fats, and potassium.

6. Veggie Breakfast Burrito:

Ingredients:

Tortilla, scrambled eggs, black beans, bell peppers, onions, salsa, cheese.

Preparation:

Fill a tortilla with scrambled eggs, black beans, bell peppers, onions, salsa, and cheese. Roll it up.

Prep Time:

15 minutes

Nutritional Value:

High in protein, fiber, and vitamins.

7. Fruit Salad:

Ingredients:

Assorted fruits (strawberries, blueberries, grapes, melon, etc.), lemon juice, honey, mint leaves (optional).

Preparation:

Cut fruits into bite-sized pieces. Toss with lemon juice and honey. Garnish with mint leaves if desired.

Prep Time:

10 minutes

Nutritional Value:

Packed with vitamins, antioxidants, and fiber.

8. Breakfast Quinoa:

Ingredients:

Quinoa, milk (or water), honey, nuts, dried fruits.

Preparation:

Cook quinoa in milk/water until tender. Sweeten with honey. Top with nuts and dried fruits.

Prep Time:

20 minutes

Nutritional Value:

Maximum in fiber, vital minerals, and protein.

9. Whole Grain Pancakes:

Ingredients:

Whole wheat flour, milk, eggs, baking powder, honey, vanilla extract.

Preparation:

Combine all ingredients in a bowl. Mix until smooth. Cook pancakes on a greased griddle.

Prep Time:

15 minutes

Nutritional Value:

Good source of fiber and nutrients.

10. Breakfast Muffins:

Ingredients:

Eggs, vegetables (spinach, tomatoes, mushrooms, etc.), cheese, salt, pepper.

Preparation:

Beat eggs with salt and pepper. Add sautéed vegetables and cheese. Pour into muffin tins. Bake until set.

Prep Time:

20 minutes

Nutritional Value:

High in protein and vitamins.

Lunch

1. Grilled Chicken Salad:

Ingredients:

- Grilled chicken breast

- Mixed salad greens

- Cherry tomatoes

- Cucumber

- Red onion

- Avocado

- Olive oil

- Lemon juice

- Salt and pepper

Preparation:

1. Season the chicken breast with salt and pepper, then grill until cooked.

2. Chop the salad greens, cherry tomatoes, cucumber, red onion, and avocado.

3. In a dish, combine the salad greens, vegetables, and sliced grilled chicken.

4. Drizzle with olive oil and lemon juice, then season with salt and pepper to taste.

Prep Time:

20 minutes

Nutritional Value:

High in protein, vitamins, and healthy fats.

2. Caprese Sandwich:

Ingredients:

- Ciabatta bread

- Fresh mozzarella cheese

- Tomato

- Fresh basil leaves

- Balsamic glaze

- Salt and pepper

Preparation:

1. Slice the ciabatta bread in half.

2. Layer slices of fresh mozzarella cheese, tomato, and basil leaves on the bread.

3. Add salt and pepper and drizzle with balsamic glaze.

4. Press the sandwich together and cut into halves or quarters.

Prep Time:

10 minutes

Nutritional Value:

Source of calcium, vitamins, and antioxidants.

3. Quinoa Salad:

Ingredients:

- Cooked quinoa

- Mixture of vegetables that includes bell peppers, peas, and carrots

- Red onion

- Fresh parsley

- Olive oil

- Lemon juice

- Salt and pepper

Preparation:

1. Prepare the quinoa in accordance with the package directions, then let it cool.

2. Chop the mixed vegetables, red onion, and fresh parsley.

3. In a bowl, combine the cooked quinoa, vegetables, red onion, and parsley.

4. Drizzle with olive oil and lemon juice, then season with salt and pepper to taste.

Prep Time: 15 minutes

Nutritional Value:

High in fiber, protein, and vitamins.

4. Tuna Wrap:

Ingredients:

- Canned tuna

- Whole wheat tortilla

- Greek yogurt

- Dijon mustard

- Lettuce

- Tomato

- Cucumber

- Salt and pepper

Preparation:

1. Drain the canned tuna and place it in a bowl.

2. Mix with Greek yogurt, Dijon mustard, salt, and pepper.

3. Place the tuna mixture on a whole wheat tortilla.

4. Top with lettuce, tomato, and cucumber.

5. Roll up the tortilla tightly and cut into halves or quarters.

Prep Time:

10 minutes

Nutritional Value:

Abundant in vitamins, omega-3 fatty acids, and protein.

5. Chickpea Salad:

Ingredients:

- Canned chickpeas

- Cherry tomatoes

- Cucumber

- Red onion

- Fresh parsley

- Olive oil

- Lemon juice

- Salt and pepper

Preparation:

1. Rinse and drain the canned chickpeas.

2. Chop the cherry tomatoes, cucumber, red onion, and fresh parsley.

3. In a bowl, combine chickpeas, vegetables, red onion, and parsley.

4. Drizzle with olive oil and lemon juice, then season with salt and pepper to taste.

Prep Time:

10 minutes

Nutritional Value:

High in protein, fiber, and vitamins.

6. Turkey and Avocado Wrap:

Ingredients:

- Sliced turkey breast

- Whole wheat tortilla

- Avocado

- Lettuce

- Tomato

- Greek yogurt

- Salt and pepper

Preparation:

1. Spread Greek yogurt on a whole wheat tortilla.

2. Layer slices of turkey breast, avocado, lettuce, and tomato on the tortilla.

3. Sprinkle with salt and pepper.

4. Roll up the tortilla tightly and cut into halves or quarters.

Prep Time:

10 minutes

Nutritional Value:

High in protein, healthy fats, and vitamins

7. Lentil Soup:

Ingredients:

- Red lentils

- Carrots

- Celery

- Onion

- Garlic

- Vegetable broth

- Cumin

- Paprika

- Salt and pepper

Preparation:

1. Rinse the red lentils, then reserve them.

2. Chop the carrots, celery, onion, and garlic.

3. In a pot, sauté the vegetables until they soften.

4. Add the red lentils, vegetable broth, cumin, paprika, salt, and pepper to the pot.

5. Simmer until the lentils are tender.

Prep Time:

30 minutes

Nutritional Value:

High in fiber, vitamins, and minerals, as well as protein.

8. Chicken Stir-Fry:

Ingredients:

- Chicken breast

- Mixed vegetables (such as bell peppers, broccoli, and snap peas)

- Soy sauce

- Garlic

- Ginger

- Olive oil

- Salt and pepper

Preparation:

1. Make thin strips out of the chicken breast.

2. Chop the mixed vegetables, garlic, and ginger.

3. In a pan, heat olive oil and sauté the chicken until cooked through.

4. Add the mixed vegetables, garlic, and ginger to the pan, and cook until tender.

5. Drizzle with soy sauce and season with salt and pepper to taste.

Prep Time:

20 minutes

Nutritional Value:

Very high in protein, fiber, and a range of vitamins and minerals.

9. Spinach and Feta Salad:

Ingredients:

- Baby spinach

- Feta cheese

- Cherry tomatoes

- Red onion

- Kalamata olives

- Olive oil

- Lemon juice

- Salt and pepper

Preparation:

1. Cleanse and pat the young spinach leaves dry.

2. Chop the feta cheese, cherry tomatoes, red onion, and Kalamata olives.

3. In a bowl, combine the baby spinach, feta cheese, cherry tomatoes, red onion, and Kalamata olives.

4. Drizzle with olive oil and lemon juice, then season with salt and pepper to taste.

Prep Time:

10 minutes

Nutritional Value:

High in vitamins, calcium, and healthy fats.

10. Veggie Wrap:

Ingredients:

- Whole wheat tortilla

- Hummus

- Avocado

- Cucumber

- Bell peppers

- Spinach leaves

- Salt and pepper

Preparation:

1. Spread hummus on a whole wheat tortilla.

2. Slice the avocado, cucumber, and bell peppers.

3. Place the sliced avocado, cucumber, bell peppers, and spinach leaves on the tortilla.

4. Sprinkle with salt and pepper.

5. Roll up the tortilla tightly and cut into halves or quarters.

Prep Time:

10 minutes

Nutritional Value:

High in fiber, vitamins, and healthy fats.

Dinner

1. Lemon Garlic Salmon:

Ingredients:

Salmon fillets, lemon juice, garlic cloves, olive oil, salt, pepper.

Preparation:

Preheat oven to 400°F. Place salmon fillets on a baking sheet. Drizzle with lemon juice, minced garlic, and olive oil. Sprinkle with salt and pepper. Bake for 12-15 minutes.

Prep Time:

20 minutes.

Nutritional Value:

High in protein and omega-3 fatty acids.

2. Chicken Stir-Fry:

Ingredients:

Chicken breast, mixed vegetables (broccoli, bell peppers, carrots), soy sauce, garlic, ginger, sesame oil.

Preparation:

Heat oil in a pan add chicken, garlic, and ginger. Cook until chicken is browned. Add vegetables and stir-fry until tender. Mix in soy sauce and cook for a few more minutes.

Prep Time:

25 minutes.

Nutritional Value:

High in protein, fiber, and vitamins.

3. Quinoa Salad:

Ingredients:

Quinoa, cucumbers, cherry tomatoes, red onion, feta cheese, olive oil, lemon juice, fresh herbs (such as parsley or basil).

Preparation:

Cook quinoa according to package instructions. Chop cucumbers, cherry tomatoes, and red onion. In a bowl, combine cooked quinoa, vegetables, feta cheese, olive oil, lemon juice, and herbs. Toss well.

Prep Time:

30 minutes.

Nutritional Value:

High in fiber, protein, and antioxidants.

4. Shrimp Scampi:

Ingredients:

Shrimp, garlic, butter, lemon juice, white wine, parsley, salt, pepper.

Preparation:

In a skillet, melt butter and sauté garlic until fragrant. Add shrimp and cook. Add salt, pepper, white wine, parsley, and lemon juice until pink. Cook for a few more minutes.

Prep Time:

20 minutes.

Nutritional Value:

High in protein and healthy fats.

5. Veggie Stir-Fry:

Ingredients:

Assorted vegetables (such as bell peppers, broccoli, carrots, snap peas), garlic, soy sauce, sesame oil.

Preparation:

Garlic is cooked until aromatic in hot oil in a pan. Add vegetables and stir-fry until tender. Mix in soy sauce and cook for a few more minutes.

Prep Time:

20 minutes.

Nutritional Value:

High in fiber, vitamins, and minerals.

6. Baked Chicken Parmesan:

Ingredients:

Chicken breast, marinara sauce, mozzarella cheese, Parmesan cheese, breadcrumbs, Italian seasoning.

Preparation:

Preheat oven to 400°F. Coat chicken breast with breadcrumbs and Italian seasoning. Place on a baking sheet and bake for 20-25 minutes. Top with marinara sauce and cheese. Bake until cheese melts.

Prep Time:

30 minutes.

Nutritional Value:

High in protein and calcium.

7. Lentil Soup:

Ingredients:

Lentils, vegetable broth, carrots, celery, onion, garlic, cumin, paprika, salt, pepper.

Preparation:

Sauté the celery, carrots, onion, and garlic in a saucepan. Add lentils, vegetable broth, cumin, paprika, salt, and pepper. Simmer until lentils are tender.

Prep Time:

40 minutes.

Nutritional Value:

High in fiber, protein, and iron.

8. Spinach and Feta Stuffed Chicken:

Ingredients: Chicken breast, spinach, feta cheese, garlic, olive oil, salt, pepper.

Preparation:

Preheat oven to 375°F. Butterfly chicken breast. In a bowl, mix spinach, feta cheese, garlic, salt, and pepper. Spread mixture on one side of the chicken breast. Fold over and secure with toothpicks. Bake for 25-30 minutes.

Prep Time:

35 minutes.

Nutritional Value:

High in protein, calcium, and vitamins.

9. Beef and Broccoli Stir-Fry:

Ingredients:

Beef, broccoli florets, soy sauce, garlic, ginger, brown sugar, cornstarch, sesame oil.

Preparation:

In a pan, stir-fry beef until browned. Add garlic and ginger. Add broccoli and cook until tender. In a bowl, mix soy sauce, brown sugar, cornstarch, and water. When the sauce is added, stir it around to combine.

Prep Time:

 25 minutes.

Nutritional Value:

High in protein, fiber, and vitamins.

10. Veggie Wrap:

Ingredients:

Tortilla wrap, hummus, mixed vegetables (such as lettuce, tomatoes, cucumbers, bell peppers), avocado.

Preparation:

Spread hummus on the tortilla wrap. Add mixed vegetables and sliced avocado. Slice into half or quarters after firmly rolling.

Prep Time:

10 minutes.

Nutritional Value:

High in fiber, vitamins, and healthy fats.

Snack and Dessert Recipes

1. Fruit Parfait

Ingredients:

Greek yogurt, mixed berries, granola.

Preparation:

Fill a glass with yogurt, granola, and berries.

Prep Time:

5 minutes.

Instructions: A refreshing and healthy snack packed with protein, probiotics, and antioxidants.

2. Energy Balls

Ingredients: Medjool dates, nuts, cocoa powder, shredded coconut.

Preparation:

Blend dates, nuts, and cocoa powder, roll into small balls, and coat with shredded coconut.

Prep Time:

15 minutes.

Instructions:

A sweet and satisfying snack loaded with fiber, healthy fats, and natural sugars.

3. Capresse Skewers

Ingredients:

Cherry tomatoes, fresh mozzarella, basil leaves, balsamic glaze.

Preparation:

Thread tomatoes, mozzarella, and basil leaves onto skewers, drizzle with balsamic glaze.

Prep Time:

10 minutes.

Instructions:

A savory snack that provides calcium, vitamins, and antioxidants.

4. Chocolate-Dipped Strawberries

Ingredients:

Fresh strawberries, dark chocolate.

Preparation:

Melt dark chocolate, dip strawberries in chocolate, and place on a baking sheet to set.

Prep Time:

20 minutes.

Instructions:

A sweet treat rich in antioxidants and vitamin C.

5. Cucumber Slices with Hummus

Ingredients:

Cucumber, hummus.

Preparation:

Slice cucumber into rounds, serve with hummus for dipping.

Prep Time:

5 minutes.

Instructions:

A light and refreshing snack packed with fiber, vitamins, and minerals.

6. Baked Sweet Potato Fries

Ingredients:

Sweet potatoes, olive oil, salt, paprika.

Preparation:

Cut sweet potatoes into fries, toss with olive oil, sprinkle with salt and paprika, and bake until crispy.

Prep Time:

25 minutes.

Instructions:

A healthier alternative to regular fries, providing fiber, vitamins, and antioxidants.

7. Yogurt Bark

Ingredients:

Greek yogurt, mixed berries, honey, granola.

Preparation:

Mix yogurt, berries, and honey, spread onto a baking sheet, sprinkle with granola, and freeze until firm.

Prep Time:

10 minutes.

Instructions:

A cool and creamy dessert that offers protein, probiotics and antioxidants.

8. Avocado Toast

Ingredients:

Whole grain bread, avocado, lemon juice, red pepper flakes.

Preparation:

Toast bread, mash avocado with lemon juice, spread on toast, sprinkle with red pepper flakes.

Prep Time: 5 minutes.

Instructions:

A satisfying snack rich in healthy fats, fiber, and vitamins.

9. Trail Mix

Ingredients:

Nuts, dried fruits, seeds, dark chocolate.

Preparation:

Mix nuts, dried fruits, seeds, and dark chocolate in a bowl.

Prep Time:

5 minutes.

Instructions:

A portable and nutritious snack providing protein, healthy fats, and antioxidants.

10. Apple Nachos

Ingredients:

Apples, peanut butter, granola, chocolate chips.

Preparation:

Slice apples, drizzle with peanut butter, sprinkle with granola and chocolate chips.

Prep Time:

10 minutes.

Instructions:

A fun and delicious dessert loaded with fiber, protein, and vitamins.

11. Greek Yogurt Popsicles

Ingredients:

Greek yogurt, honey, mixed berries.

Preparation:

Mix yogurt, honey, and berries, pour into popsicle molds, and freeze until solid.

Prep Time:

10 minutes.

Instructions:

A refreshing and creamy dessert packed with protein, probiotics, and antioxidants.

12. Veggie Chips

Ingredients:

Kale, sweet potatoes, olive oil, sea salt.

Preparation:

Slice kale and sweet potatoes into thin strips, toss with olive oil and sea salt, and bake until crispy.

Prep Time:

20 minutes.

Instructions:

A crunchy and nutritious snack offering vitamins, fiber, and antioxidants.

13. Banana Ice Cream

Ingredients:

Frozen bananas, almond milk, vanilla extract.

Preparation:

Blend frozen bananas, almond milk, and vanilla extract until creamy.

Prep Time:

5 minutes.

Instructions:

A guilt-free dessert that's rich in potassium, fiber, and natural sweetness.

14. Spinach and Artichoke Dip

Ingredients:

Spinach, artichoke hearts, cream cheese, Parmesan cheese.

Preparation:

Mix spinach, artichoke hearts, cream cheese, and Parmesan cheese, and bake until bubbly.

Prep Time:

15 minutes.

Instructions:

A creamy and flavorful dip that provides calcium, vitamins, and antioxidants.

15. Popcorn with Dark Chocolate Drizzle

Ingredients:

Popcorn, dark chocolate.

Preparation:

Pop popcorn, melt dark chocolate, drizzle over popcorn.

Prep Time:

10 minutes.

Instructions:

A sweet and crunchy snack with whole grains, antioxidants, and fiber.

16. Banana Sushi

Ingredients:

Banana, nut butter, granola.

Preparation:

Slice banana, spread with nut butter, roll in granola.

Prep Time:

5 minutes.

Instructions:

A fun and nutritious snack offering potassium, healthy fats, and fiber.

17. Mini Quiches

Ingredients:

Eggs, vegetables, cheese, spices.

Preparation:

Whisk eggs, mix in vegetables, cheese, and spices, pour into muffin tins, and bake until set.

Prep Time:

15 minutes.

Instructions:

A protein-packed snack with vitamins, minerals, and flavor.

18. Frozen Grapes

Ingredients:

Grapes.

Preparation:

Freeze grapes until firm.

Prep Time:

5 minutes.

Instructions:

A simple and refreshing snack with natural sugars and antioxidants.

19. Peanut Butter Banana Bites

Ingredients:

Bananas, peanut butter, dark chocolate.

Preparation:

Slice bananas, spread with peanut butter, sandwich with another banana slice, dip in melted dark chocolate.

Prep Time:

10 minutes.

Instructions:

A decadent and nutritious dessert offering potassium, protein, and antioxidants.

20. Rice Cake with Nutella and Berries

Ingredients: Rice cakes, Nutella, mixed berries.

Preparation:

Spread Nutella on rice cakes, top with mixed berries.

Prep Time:

5 minutes.

Instructions:

A sweet and crunchy snack that provides fiber, antioxidants, and a touch of indulgence.

Nourishing Soups and Stews

1. Lentil Soup:

Ingredients:

Lentils, onions, carrots, celery, vegetable broth, garlic, cumin, turmeric, salt, pepper.

Preparation:

Sauté onions, carrots, and celery. Add lentils, broth, and spices. Simmer for 30 minutes.

Prep Time:

40 minutes.

Nutritional Value:

High in fiber, protein, and iron.

2. Chicken Noodle Soup:

Ingredients:

Chicken breast, egg noodles, carrots, celery, chicken broth, garlic, parsley, salt, pepper.

Preparation:

Cook chicken, shred it, and set aside. Sauté carrots, celery, and garlic. Add broth, noodles, and chicken. Simmer until noodles are cooked.

Prep Time:

45 minutes.

Nutritional Value:

Good source of protein and vitamins.

3. Vegetable Minestrone:

Ingredients:

Onion, garlic, carrots, celery, zucchini, tomatoes, kidney beans, vegetable broth, pasta, basil, oregano, salt, pepper.

Preparation:

Sauté onion, garlic, carrots, celery, and zucchini. Add tomatoes, beans, broth, and spices. Simmer for 20 minutes.

Prep Time:

40 minutes.

Nutritional Value:

Packed with vegetables, fiber, and antioxidants.

4. Beef Stew:

Ingredients:

Beef chunks, potatoes, carrots, onions, garlic, beef broth, tomato paste, Worcestershire sauce, thyme, rosemary, salt, pepper.

Preparation:

Brown beef, set aside. Sauté onions, garlic, carrots, and potatoes. Add beef, broth, tomato paste, and spices. Simmer for 1 hour.

Prep Time:

1 hour 30 minutes.

Nutritional Value:

Rich in protein, vitamins, and minerals.

5. Tomato Basil Soup:

Ingredients:

Tomatoes, onions, garlic, vegetable broth, basil, olive oil, salt, pepper.

Preparation:

Sauté onions and garlic. Add tomatoes, broth, basil, and spices. Simmer for 20 minutes.

Prep Time:

30 minutes.

Nutritional Value:

High in antioxidants and vitamins.

6. Butternut Squash Soup:

Ingredients:

Butternut squash, onion, garlic, vegetable broth, coconut milk, nutmeg, cinnamon, salt, pepper.

Preparation:

Roast butternut squash. Sauté onion and garlic. Blend squash, onion, garlic, broth, coconut milk, and spices. Heat until warm.

Prep Time:

1 hour.

Nutritional Value:

Rich in vitamins A and C, fiber, and antioxidants.

7. Black Bean Soup:

Ingredients:

Black beans, onion, garlic, vegetable broth, cumin, paprika, chili powder, lime juice, cilantro, salt, pepper.

Preparation:

Sauté onion and garlic. Add beans, broth, spices, and lime juice. Simmer for 30 minutes.

Prep Time:

40 minutes.

Nutritional Value:

High in fiber, protein, and antioxidants.

8. Chicken Tortilla Soup:

Ingredients:

Chicken breast, onion, garlic, tomatoes, black beans, corn, chicken broth, cumin, chili powder, lime juice, cilantro, salt, pepper.

Preparation:

Cook chicken, shred it. Sauté onion and garlic. Add tomatoes, beans, corn, broth, spices, and lime juice. Simmer for 20 minutes.

Prep Time:

45 minutes.

Nutritional Value:

Good source of protein and fiber.

9. Moroccan Chickpea Stew:

Ingredients:

Chickpeas, onion, garlic, tomatoes, carrots, vegetable broth, cumin, paprika, turmeric, cinnamon, salt, pepper.

Preparation:

Sauté onion and garlic. Add chickpeas, tomatoes, carrots, broth, and spices. Simmer for 30 minutes.

Prep Time:

40 minutes.

Nutritional Value:

High in fiber, protein, and antioxidants.

10. Creamy Mushroom Soup:

Ingredients:

Mushrooms, onion, garlic, vegetable broth, coconut milk, thyme, rosemary, salt, pepper.

Preparation:

Sauté onion and garlic. Add mushrooms, broth, coconut milk, and spices. Simmer for 20 minutes.

Prep Time:

30 minutes.

Nutritional Value:

Low in calories, high in vitamins and minerals.

11. Spinach and White Bean Soup:

Ingredients:

White beans, spinach, onion, garlic, vegetable broth, lemon juice, thyme, salt, pepper.

Preparation:

Sauté onion and garlic. Add beans, spinach, broth, lemon juice, and spices. Simmer for 15 minutes.

Prep Time:

25 minutes.

Nutritional Value:

High in fiber, iron, and vitamins.

12. Thai Coconut Curry Soup:

Ingredients:

Coconut milk, vegetable broth, curry paste, tofu, mushrooms, bell peppers, carrots, lime juice, cilantro, salt, pepper.

Preparation:

Heat coconut milk, broth, and curry paste. Add tofu, mushrooms, bell peppers, carrots, lime juice, and spices. Simmer for 20 minutes.

Prep Time:

40 minutes.

Nutritional Value:

Rich in protein, vitamins, and healthy fats.

13. Chicken and Rice Soup:

Ingredients:

Chicken breast, rice, carrots, celery, onion, garlic, chicken broth, thyme, parsley, salt, pepper.

Preparation:

Cook chicken, shred it. Sauté carrots, celery, onion, and garlic. Add chicken, rice, broth, and spices. Simmer until rice is cooked.

Prep Time:

50 minutes.

Nutritional Value:

Good source of protein and carbohydrates.

14. Italian Wedding Soup:

Ingredients:

Meatballs, spinach, onion, garlic, carrots, celery, chicken broth, pasta, parsley, salt, pepper.

Preparation:

Sauté onion, garlic, carrots, and celery. Add meatballs, spinach, broth, pasta, and spices. Simmer for 20 minutes.

Prep Time:

40 minutes.

Nutritional Value:

High in protein, vitamins, and minerals.

15. Potato Leek Soup:

Ingredients:

Potatoes, leeks, onion, garlic, vegetable broth, thyme, bay leaf, salt, pepper.

Preparation:

Sauté leeks, onion, and garlic. Add potatoes, broth, and spices. Simmer until potatoes are tender. Blend until smooth.

Prep Time:

45 minutes.

Nutritional Value:

Good source of potassium, vitamin C, and fiber.

16. Corn Chowder:

Ingredients:

Corn, potatoes, onion, garlic, vegetable broth, milk, thyme, paprika, salt, pepper.

Preparation:

Sauté onion and garlic. Add corn, potatoes, broth, milk, and spices. Simmer for 30 minutes.

Prep Time:

50 minutes.

Nutritional Value:

High in fiber, vitamins, and minerals.

17. Red Lentil Curry Soup:

Ingredients:

Red lentils, onion, garlic, tomatoes, coconut milk, curry powder, cumin, paprika, turmeric, salt, pepper.

Preparation:

Sauté onion and garlic. Add lentils, tomatoes, coconut milk, and spices. Simmer until lentils are cooked.

Prep Time:

40 minutes.

Nutritional Value:

Rich in protein, fiber, and antioxidants.

18. Mexican Tortilla Soup:

Ingredients:

Tomatoes, onion, garlic, vegetable broth, corn, black beans, chili powder, cumin, lime juice, cilantro, salt, pepper.

Preparation:

Sauté onion and garlic. Add tomatoes, broth, corn, beans, spices, and lime juice. Simmer for 20 minutes.

Prep Time:

40 minutes.

Nutritional Value:

High in fiber, vitamins, and minerals.

19. Clam Chowder:

Ingredients:

Clams, potatoes, onion, garlic, bacon, milk, vegetable broth, thyme, parsley, salt, pepper.

Preparation:

Sauté onion, garlic, and bacon. Add clams, potatoes, broth, milk, and spices. Simmer until potatoes are tender.

Prep Time:

1 hour.

Nutritional Value:

Good source of protein and vitamins.

20. Moroccan Harira Soup:

Ingredients:

Lentils, chickpeas, onion, garlic, tomatoes, celery, parsley, cilantro, cinnamon, turmeric, ginger, salt, pepper.

Preparation:

Sauté onion, garlic, celery, and spices. Add lentils, chickpeas, tomatoes, and water. Simmer for 1 hour.

Prep Time:

1 hour 15 minutes.

Nutritional Value:

High in fiber, protein, and antioxidants.

Sauce

1. Marinara Sauce:

Ingredients:

- 1 can (28 oz) crushed tomatoes

- 2 cloves garlic, minced

- 2 tablespoons olive oil

- 1 teaspoon dried oregano

- Salt and pepper to taste

Preparation:

1. Heat olive oil in a saucepan, sauté garlic until fragrant.

2. Add the oregano, smashed tomatoes, salt, and pepper.

3. Simmer for 15-20 minutes.

Prep Time:

25 minutes

Nutritional Value:

Approximately 80 calories per 1/2 cup serving.

2. Pesto Sauce:

Ingredients:

- 2 cups fresh basil leaves

- 1/2 cup grated Parmesan cheese

- 1/2 cup pine nuts

- 2 cloves garlic

- 1/2 cup olive oil

- Salt and pepper to taste

Preparation:

Put all the ingredients in a food processor and pulse until smooth.

Prep Time:

10 minutes

Nutritional Value:

Approximately 250 calories per 1/4 cup serving.

3. Teriyaki Sauce:

Ingredients:

- 1/2 cup soy sauce

- 1/4 cup brown sugar

- 2 cloves garlic, minced

- 1 tablespoon grated ginger

- 1 tablespoon cornstarch (optional)

Preparation:

1. Combine all ingredients in a saucepan.

2. Heat and stir until it thickens (add cornstarch if desired).

Prep Time:

10 minutes

Nutritional Value:

Approximately 40 calories per 2-tablespoon serving.

4. Alfredo Sauce:

- Ingredients:

- 1 cup heavy cream

- 1/2 cup unsalted butter

- 1 cup grated Parmesan cheese

- 2 cloves garlic, minced

- Salt and pepper to taste

Preparation:

1. Melt butter in a saucepan, add garlic and cook briefly.

2. Add heavy cream and Parmesan cheese, and stir.

3. Season with salt and pepper.

Prep Time:

15 minutes

Nutritional Value:

Approximately 350 calories per 1/4 cup serving.

5. Salsa:

Ingredients:

- 3 ripe tomatoes, diced

- 1/2 onion, finely chopped

- 1 jalapeño, seeded and minced

- 2 cloves garlic, minced

- 2 tablespoons fresh lime juice

- Salt and pepper to taste

Preparation:

1. Combine all ingredients in a bowl.

Prep Time:

10 minutes

Nutritional Value:

Approximately 15 calories per 1/4 cup serving.

6. Hollandaise Sauce:

Ingredients:

- 3 egg yolks

- 1 tablespoon lemon juice

- 1/2 cup unsalted butter

- Cayenne pepper, to taste

Preparation:

1. Melt butter in a saucepan, set aside.

2. In a blender, combine egg yolks and lemon juice.

3. Slowly add melted butter while blending.

4. Season with cayenne pepper.

Prep Time:

15 minutes

Nutritional Value:

Approximately 90 calories per 2 tablespoon serving.

7. BBQ Sauce:

Ingredients:

- 1 cup ketchup

- 1/4 cup brown sugar

- 2 tablespoons vinegar

- 1 tablespoon Worcestershire sauce

- 1 teaspoon smoked paprika

- 1/2 teaspoon garlic powder

Preparation:

1. Mix all ingredients in a saucepan and simmer for 10 minutes.

Prep Time:

15 minutes

Nutritional Value:

Approximately 60 calories per 2 tablespoon serving.

8. Chimichurri Sauce:

Ingredients:

- 1 cup fresh parsley, chopped

- 1/4 cup red wine vinegar

- 3 cloves garlic, minced

- 1/2 cup olive oil

- 1 teaspoon red pepper flakes

- Salt and pepper to taste

Preparation:

1. Combine all ingredients in a bowl.

Prep Time:

10 minutes

Nutritional Value:

Approximately 150 calories per 2 tablespoon serving.

9. Thai Peanut Sauce:

Ingredients:

- 1/2 cup peanut butter

- 2 tablespoons soy sauce

- 2 tablespoons lime juice

- 2 tablespoons honey

- 1 clove garlic, minced

- 1/2 teaspoon red pepper flakes (optional)

Preparation:

1. Blend every component in a bowl by whisking them together.

Prep Time:

10 minutes

Nutritional Value:

Approximately 90 calories per 2 tablespoon serving.

10. Lemon Butter Sauce:

Ingredients:

- 1/2 cup unsalted butter

- 2 tablespoons lemon juice

- 1 teaspoon lemon zest

- 2 cloves garlic, minced

- Salt and pepper to taste

Preparation:

1. Melt butter in a saucepan, add garlic and cook briefly.

2. Stir in lemon juice and zest.

3. Season with salt and pepper.

Prep Time:

10 minutes

Nutritional Value:

Approximately 140 calories per 2-tablespoon serving.

1. Classic Strawberry Banana Smoothie:

Ingredients:

- 1 cup strawberries, frozen

- 1 ripe banana

- 1/2 cup Greek yogurt

- One-half cup milk (or substitute)

- 1 tablespoon honey (optional)

Preparation:

1. Combine all ingredients in a blender.

2. Blend until well mixed

Prep Time:

5 minutes

Nutritional Value:

Approximately 250 calories per serving.

2. Green Spinach and Mango Smoothie:

- Ingredients:

- 1 cup baby spinach leaves

- 1 cup frozen mango chunks

- 1/2 cup Greek yogurt

- 1/2 cup water or coconut water

- 1 tablespoon honey (optional)

Preparation:

1. Blend all ingredients in a blender until smooth.

Prep Time:

5 minutes

Nutritional Value:

Approximately 200 calories per serving.

3. Blueberry and Almond Butter Smoothie:

Ingredients:

- 1/2 cup blueberries, frozen

- 1 tablespoon almond butter

- 1/2 cup Greek yogurt

- 1/2 cup almond milk

- 1 teaspoon honey (optional)

Preparation:

1. Combine all ingredients in a blender.

2. Blend until well mixed.

Prep Time:

5 minutes

Nutritional Value:

Approximately 220 calories per serving.

4. Chocolate Banana Protein Smoothie:

Ingredients:

- 1 ripe banana

- 2 tablespoons cocoa powder

- 1/2 cup Greek yogurt

- One-half cup milk (or substitute)

- One scoop of your preferred protein powder

Preparation:

1. Blend all ingredients in a blender until creamy.

Prep Time:

5 minutes

Nutritional Value:

Approximately 300 calories per serving.

5. Tropical Pineapple and Coconut Smoothie:

Ingredients:

- 1 cup pineapple chunks, frozen

- 1/2 cup coconut milk

- 1/2 cup Greek yogurt

- 1/4 cup orange juice

- 1 tablespoon honey (optional)

Preparation:

1. Blend all ingredients in a blender until smooth.

Prep Time:

5 minutes

Nutritional Value:

Approximately 260 calories per serving.

6. Peanut Butter and Banana Smoothie:

Ingredients:

- 1 ripe banana

- 2 tablespoons peanut butter

- 1/2 cup Greek yogurt

- One-half cup milk (or substitute)

- 1 teaspoon honey (optional)

Preparation:

1. Blend all ingredients in a blender until well combined.

Prep Time:

5 minutes

Nutritional Value:

Approximately 280 calories per serving.

7. Raspberry and Kale Smoothie:

- Ingredients:

- 1/2 cup frozen raspberries

- 1 cup kale leaves

- 1/2 cup Greek yogurt

- 1/2 cup water or almond milk

- 1 tablespoon honey (optional)

Preparation:

1. Blend all ingredients in a blender until smooth.

Prep Time:

5 minutes

Nutritional Value:

Approximately 190 calories per serving.

8. Oatmeal and Apple Cinnamon Smoothie:

Ingredients:

- 1/2 cup rolled oats

- 1 apple, peeled and chopped

- 1/2 teaspoon ground cinnamon

- 1/2 cup Greek yogurt

- 1/2 cup milk (or a milk alternative)

Preparation:

1. Combine all ingredients in a blender and blend until creamy.

Prep Time:

7 minutes (includes soaking oats)

Nutritional Value:

Approximately 290 calories per serving.

9. Avocado and Spinach Smoothie:

Ingredients:

- 1/2 avocado

- 1 cup baby spinach leaves

- 1/2 cup Greek yogurt

- 1/2 cup water or coconut water

- 1 tablespoon honey (optional)

Preparation:

1. Blend all ingredients in a blender until smooth.

Prep Time:

5 minutes

Nutritional Value:

Approximately 230 calories per serving.

10. Cherry and Chia Seed Smoothie:

Ingredients:

- 1 cup cherries, frozen

- 1 tablespoon chia seeds

- 1/2 cup Greek yogurt

- 1/2 cup almond milk

- 1 teaspoon honey (optional)

Preparation:

1. Blend all ingredients in a blender until well-mixed.

Prep Time:

5 minutes

Nutritional Value:

Approximately 240 calories per serving.

Time-saving kitchen Hacks For Weight Loss

1. Pre-Pack Smoothie Bags:

- Kitchen Hack: Pre-pack your smoothie ingredients in freezer bags for a quick morning blend.

- Recipe: In a bag, combine frozen berries, spinach, a banana, a tablespoon of chia seeds, and almond milk. Blend when ready.

- Weight Loss Tip: Smoothies can be packed with nutrients and low in calories if you skip added sugars.

2. Sheet Pan Meals:

- Kitchen Hack: Use sheet pans to roast a variety of veggies and lean protein simultaneously.

- Recipe: Place chicken breast, broccoli, and sweet potatoes on a sheet pan. Drizzle with olive oil and season. Roast at 400°F (200°C) for 25-30 minutes.

- Weight Loss Tip: Sheet pan meals are easy to portion and control serving sizes.

3. Overnight Oats:

- Kitchen Hack: Prep a week's worth of overnight oats in advance.

- Recipe: Combine oats, almond milk, chia seeds, and your choice of sweetener. Refrigerate overnight and top with fruits in the morning.

- Weight Loss Tip: Oats are fiber-rich, which helps control appetite.

4. Mason Jar Salads:

- Kitchen Hack: Prepare salads in mason jars for grab-and-go lunches.

- Recipe: Layer your favorite salad ingredients in a jar, starting with dressing at the bottom and greens at the top.

- Weight Loss Tip: Controlling portion sizes and ingredients in advance can help with mindful eating.

5. One-Pot Pasta:

- Kitchen Hack: Cook pasta and sauce in one pot to save time and cleanup.

- Recipe: Combine whole wheat pasta, cherry tomatoes, garlic, olive oil, and a pinch of red pepper flakes in a pot. Add boiled water and simmer until the pasta is tender.

- Weight Loss Tip: Whole wheat pasta and fresh tomatoes make this a healthier option.

6. Protein-Packed Stir-Fry:

- Kitchen Hack: Use pre-cut veggies and lean protein for a quick stir-fry.

- Recipe: Stir-fry diced chicken breast, mixed vegetables, and a low-sodium stir-fry sauce.

- Weight Loss Tip: Lean protein and vegetables make a filling, low-calorie meal.

7. Chia Pudding:

- Kitchen Hack: Mix chia seeds with almond milk the night before for a quick breakfast.

- Recipe: Combine chia seeds and almond milk in a jar, and add a touch of honey and vanilla. Refrigerate overnight and top with berries.

- Weight Loss Tip: Chia seeds are high in fiber and protein.

8. Veggie Omelet:

- Kitchen Hack: Use a non-stick skillet for a quick health omelet.

- Recipe: Whisk eggs, pour into a heated skillet, add diced veggies, and fold the omelet in half.

- Weight Loss Tip: Eggs are a protein-packed option for breakfast or lunch.

9. Instant Pot Quinoa:

- Kitchen Hack: Use an Instant Pot for quick and perfect quinoa.

- Recipe: Combine quinoa, water, and a pinch of salt in the Instant Pot. Manually put it for one minute, then allow a natural release for 10 minutes.

- Weight Loss Tip: Quinoa is a nutritious and filling grain.

10. DIY Salad Dressings:

- Kitchen Hack: Make your salad dressings for healthier salads.

- Recipe: Combine olive oil, vinegar, mustard, honey, and herbs and spices.

- Weight Loss Tip: Homemade dressings allow you to control the ingredients and avoid excess sugars.

These time-saving kitchen hacks and weight loss recipes can help you eat healthy while making the most of your busy schedule.

CHAPTER 5

Exercises for weight loss

1. Jacks: Start with your feet together and your arms at your sides. Jump your feet to the side and raise your arms above your head. Jump back to the starting position. Repeat for 1 minute.

2. Squats: Stand with your feet shoulder-width apart and your arms at your sides. Lower your body as if you were sitting in a chair, keeping your back straight and your knees behind your toes. Push back up to the starting position. Repeat for 1 minute.

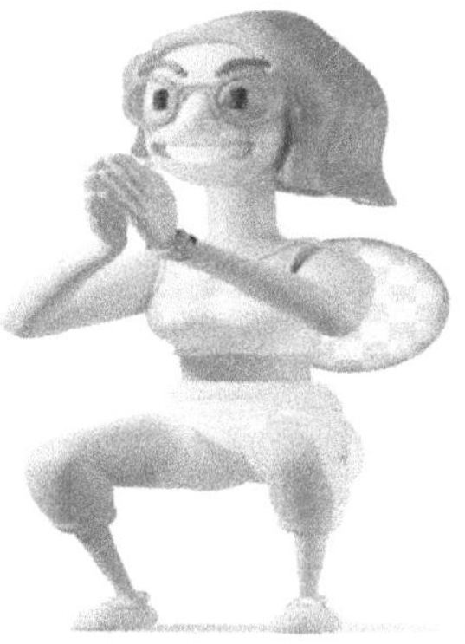

3. Push-ups: Start in a plank position with your hands slightly wider than shoulder-width apart. Lower your body until your chest

nearly touches the floor. Push back up to the starting position. Repeat for 1 minute.

4. Burpees: Start in a standing position. Squat down and place your hands on the floor. Jump your feet back into a plank position. Jump your feet back up to your hands and stand up. Repeat for 1 minute.

5. Mountain climbers: Start in a plank position with your hands slightly wider than shoulder-width apart. Bring one knee up towards your chest and then switch legs. Repeat for 1 minute.

6. Jump rope: Start with your feet together and your arms at your sides. Jump over the rope as it passes under your feet. Repeat for 1 minute.

7. Lunges: Stand with your feet shoulder-width apart and your arms at your sides. Step forward with one leg and lower your body until your back knee nearly touches the floor. Push back up to the starting position. Repeat for 1 minute.

8. Plank: Start in a plank position with your hands slightly wider than shoulder-width apart. Hold this position for 1 minute.

9. High knees: Start with your feet together and your arms at your sides. Lift one knee towards your chest and then switch legs. Repeat for 1 minute.

10. Side plank: Lie with your feet stacked and your elbow directly under your shoulder. Lift your hips off the floor and hold this position for 1 minute.

How To Stay Motivated on Your Weight Loss Journey?

1. Set realistic goals: Make sure your goals are achievable and measurable.

2. Track your progress: Keeping a record of your progress on a weight loss planner and celebrate your successes.

3. Find a support system: Surround yourself with people who will encourage and motivate you.

4. Reward yourself: Give yourself rewards for reaching milestones or sticking to your plan.

5. Exercise regularly: Exercise is an important part of any weight loss journey.

6. Eat healthy: Make sure to eat a balanced diet with plenty of fruits and vegetables.

7. Get enough sleep: Make sure you are getting enough rest to stay energized and motivated.

8. Stay positive: Don't focus on the negative, focus on the positive and what you can do to reach your goals.

9. Take breaks: Don't be too hard on yourself. Take breaks and enjoy life.

10. Believe in yourself: Believe that you can do it and you will be successful.

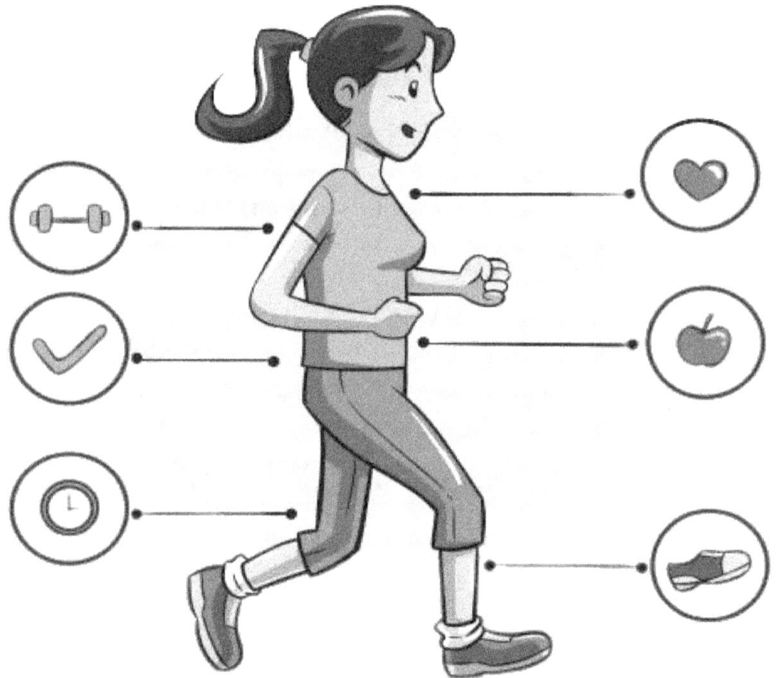

NB: Weight loss track

CONCLUSION

"Nourish and Fit" presents a unique and effective approach to weight loss through its quick and easy recipes. The book understands that in today's fast-paced world, individuals need convenient and simple solutions, and it delivers just that. The recipes provided are not only focused on weight loss but also on nourishing the body with wholesome ingredients.

The book emphasizes the importance of balance, moderation, and sustainability, with an emphasis on enjoying the process of cooking and eating. By following the recipes and guidelines in "Nourish and Fit," readers can not only achieve their weight loss goals but also develop a healthier relationship with food.

This book is an excellent resource for anyone looking to achieve weight loss practically and enjoyable without sacrificing flavor and nourishment. It is a must-read for those seeking a holistic approach to weight loss and overall well-being.

NOURISH AND FIT PLANNER

DATE: S M T W T F S

GOALS OF THE DAY

- ☐
- ☐
- ☐
- ☐

WORKHOUT	TIME	REPS

WATER

1L   2L   3L   4L

TODAY'S MOOD

DAILY NUTRITION

Breakfast

Lunch

Dinner

Snacks

TODAY'S MOTIVATION

● TO START   ✓ OK   → DELAY   ∕ STUCK   ✕ CANCEL

NOURISH AND FIT PLANNER

DATE: _______________________________ S M T W T F S

GOALS OF THE DAY

- ☐
- ☐
- ☐
- ☐

WORKHOUT	TIME	REPS
☐		
☐		
☐		
☐		
☐		
☐		
☐		
☐		
☐		
☐		
☐		
☐		
☐		
☐		
☐		

WATER

1L   2L   3L   4L

TODAY'S MOOD

DAILY NUTRITION

Breakfast

Lunch

Dinner

Snacks

TODAY'S MOTIVATION

● TO START   ✓ OK   → DELAY   ／ STUCK   ✕ CANCEL

NOURISH AND FIT PLANNER

DATE: _______________________ S M T W T F S

GOALS OF THE DAY

- [ ] _______________________
- [ ] _______________________
- [ ] _______________________
- [ ] _______________________

WORKHOUT	TIME	REPS

WATER

1L 2L 3L 4L

TODAY'S MOOD

DAILY NUTRITION

Breakfast _______________________

Lunch _______________________

Dinner _______________________

Snacks _______________________

TODAY'S MOTIVATION

____

● TO START   ✓ OK   → DELAY   / STUCK   ✗ CANCEL

NOURISH AND FIT PLANNER

DATE: ___________________________   S M T W T F S

GOALS OF THE DAY

- [ ] ________________________________
- [ ] ________________________________
- [ ] ________________________________
- [ ] ________________________________

WORKHOUT	TIME	REPS

WATER

1L   2L   3L   4L

TODAY'S MOOD

DAILY NUTRITION

Breakfast ________________________

Lunch ________________________

Dinner ________________________

Snacks ________________________

TODAY'S MOTIVATION

____

____

● TO START   ✓ OK   → DELAY   ／ STUCK   ✕ CANCEL

NOURISH AND FIT PLANNER

DATE: ___________________________ S M T W T F S

GOALS OF THE DAY

- ___________________________
- ___________________________
- ___________________________
- ___________________________

WORKHOUT	TIME	REPS

WATER

1L 2L 3L 4L

TODAY'S MOOD

DAILY NUTRITION

Breakfast ___________________

Lunch ___________________

Dinner ___________________

Snacks ___________________

TODAY'S MOTIVATION

____

____

● TO START   ✓ OK   → DELAY   ⁄ STUCK   ✕ CANCEL

NOURISH AND FIT PLANNER

DATE:

S M T W T F S

GOALS OF THE DAY

WORKHOUT | TIME | REPS

WATER

1L 2L 3L 4L

TODAY'S MOOD

DAILY NUTRITION

Breakfast

Lunch

Dinner

Snacks

TODAY'S MOTIVATION

● TO START ✓ OK → DELAY ╱ STUCK ✕ CANCEL

NOURISH AND FIT PLANNER

DATE: S   M   T   W   T   F   S

GOALS OF THE DAY

- [ ]
- [ ]
- [ ]
- [ ]

WORKHOUT	TIME	REPS
[ ]		
[ ]		
[ ]		
[ ]		
[ ]		
[ ]		
[ ]		
[ ]		
[ ]		
[ ]		
[ ]		
[ ]		
[ ]		
[ ]		

WATER

1L   2L   3L   4L

TODAY'S MOOD

DAILY NUTRITION

Breakfast

Lunch

Dinner

Snacks

TODAY'S MOTIVATION

● TO START   ✓ OK   → DELAY   ∕ STUCK   ✕ CANCEL

NOURISH AND FIT PLANNER

DATE: S M T W T F S

GOALS OF THE DAY

- ☐ ....
- ☐ ....
- ☐ ....
- ☐ ....

WORKHOUT	TIME	REPS

WATER

1L   2L   3L   4L

TODAY'S MOOD

DAILY NUTRITION

Breakfast

Lunch

Dinner

Snacks

TODAY'S MOTIVATION

● TO START   ✓ OK   → DELAY   ╱ STUCK   ✕ CANCEL

NOURISH AND FIT PLANNER

DATE: S M T W T F S

GOALS OF THE DAY

- [ ]
- [ ]
- [ ]
- [ ]

WORKHOUT	TIME	REPS

WATER

1L   2L   3L   4L

TODAY'S MOOD

DAILY NUTRITION

Breakfast

Lunch

Dinner

Snacks

TODAY'S MOTIVATION

● TO START   ✓ OK   → DELAY   ╱ STUCK   ✕ CANCEL

NOURISH AND FIT PLANNER

DATE: S M T W T F S

GOALS OF THE DAY

- [ ]
- [ ]
- [ ]
- [ ]

WORKHOUT	TIME	REPS

WATER

1L   2L   3L   4L

TODAY'S MOOD

DAILY NUTRITION

Breakfast

Lunch

Dinner

Snacks

TODAY'S MOTIVATION

● TO START   ✓ OK   → DELAY   / STUCK   ✗ CANCEL

NOURISH AND FIT PLANNER

DATE: _______________________________________ S M T W T F S

GOALS OF THE DAY

WORKHOUT   TIME   REPS

WATER

1L   2L   3L   4L

TODAY'S MOOD

DAILY NUTRITION

Breakfast _______________

Lunch _______________

Dinner _______________

Snacks _______________

TODAY'S MOTIVATION

● TO START   ✓ OK   → DELAY   ╱ STUCK   ✕ CANCEL

NOURISH AND FIT PLANNER

DATE: ___________________________   S M T W T F S

GOALS OF THE DAY

- ☐ _______________________________
- ☐ _______________________________
- ☐ _______________________________
- ☐ _______________________________

WORKHOUT	TIME	REPS
☐		
☐		
☐		
☐		
☐		
☐		
☐		
☐		
☐		
☐		
☐		
☐		
☐		
☐		
☐		

WATER

1L   2L   3L   4L

TODAY'S MOOD

DAILY NUTRITION

Breakfast _______________________

Lunch _______________________

Dinner _______________________

Snacks _______________________

TODAY'S MOTIVATION

____

● TO START   ✓ OK   → DELAY   / STUCK   ✗ CANCEL

NOURISH AND FIT PLANNER

DATE: S M T W T F S

GOALS OF THE DAY

- [ ] ________________________________
- [ ] ________________________________
- [ ] ________________________________
- [ ] ________________________________

WORKHOUT	TIME	REPS

WATER

1L   2L   3L   4L

TODAY'S MOOD

DAILY NUTRITION

Breakfast ________________________

Lunch ____________________________

Dinner ___________________________

Snacks ___________________________

TODAY'S MOTIVATION

____

____

● TO START   ✓ OK   → DELAY   ╱ STUCK   ✕ CANCEL

NOURISH AND FIT PLANNER

DATE: _______________________________________ S   M   T   W   T   F   S

GOALS OF THE DAY

- ☐ _______________________________________
- ☐ _______________________________________
- ☐ _______________________________________
- ☐ _______________________________________

WORKHOUT	TIME	REPS

WATER

1L   2L   3L   4L

TODAY'S MOOD

DAILY NUTRITION

Breakfast _______________________________

Lunch _______________________________

Dinner _______________________________

Snacks _______________________________

TODAY'S MOTIVATION

____

____

● TO START   ✓ OK   → DELAY   ⁄ STUCK   ✗ CANCEL

NOURISH AND FIT PLANNER

DATE: _______________________________ S M T W T F S

GOALS OF THE DAY

- [ ] _______________________________
- [ ] _______________________________
- [ ] _______________________________
- [ ] _______________________________

WORKHOUT	TIME	REPS

WATER

1L   2L   3L   4L

TODAY'S MOOD

DAILY NUTRITION

Breakfast _______________________

Lunch _______________________

Dinner _______________________

Snacks _______________________

TODAY'S MOTIVATION

____

____

● TO START   ✓ OK   → DELAY   ⁄ STUCK   ✕ CANCEL

NOURISH AND FIT PLANNER

DATE: S M T W T F S

GOALS OF THE DAY

- [ ]
- [ ]
- [ ]
- [ ]

WORKHOUT	TIME	REPS

WATER

1L   2L   3L   4L

TODAY'S MOOD

DAILY NUTRITION

Breakfast

Lunch

Dinner

Snacks

TODAY'S MOTIVATION

● TO START   ✓ OK   → DELAY   ／ STUCK   ✗ CANCEL

NOURISH AND FIT PLANNER

DATE: ____________________________   S M T W T F S

GOALS OF THE DAY

- [ ] ____________________________
- [ ] ____________________________
- [ ] ____________________________
- [ ] ____________________________

WORKHOUT	TIME	REPS	**WATER**

1L   2L   3L   4L

TODAY'S MOOD

DAILY NUTRITION

Breakfast ____________________

Lunch ____________________

Dinner ____________________

Snacks ____________________

TODAY'S MOTIVATION

____

____

● TO START   ✓ OK   → DELAY   ⁄ STUCK   ✗ CANCEL

NOURISH AND FIT PLANNER

DATE: S M T W T F S

GOALS OF THE DAY

WORKHOUT   TIME   REPS

WATER

1L   2L   3L   4L

TODAY'S MOOD

DAILY NUTRITION

Breakfast

Lunch

Dinner

Snacks

TODAY'S MOTIVATION

● TO START   ✓ OK   → DELAY   ╱ STUCK   ✕ CANCEL

NOURISH AND FIT PLANNER

DATE: S M T W T F S

GOALS OF THE DAY

- [ ]
- [ ]
- [ ]
- [ ]

WORKHOUT	TIME	REPS

WATER

1L   2L   3L   4L

TODAY'S MOOD

DAILY NUTRITION

Breakfast

Lunch

Dinner

Snacks

TODAY'S MOTIVATION

● TO START   ✓ OK   → DELAY   ⁄ STUCK   ✕ CANCEL

NOURISH AND FIT PLANNER

DATE: S M T W T F S

GOALS OF THE DAY

WORKHOUT   TIME   REPS   **WATER**

1L   2L   3L   4L

TODAY'S MOOD

DAILY NUTRITION

Breakfast

Lunch

Dinner

Snacks

TODAY'S MOTIVATION

● TO START   ✓ OK   → DELAY   ╱ STUCK   ✕ CANCEL

NOURISH AND FIT PLANNER

DATE: ________________________________ S M T W T F S

GOALS OF THE DAY

- [ ] _______________________________________
- [ ] _______________________________________
- [ ] _______________________________________
- [ ] _______________________________________

WORKHOUT	TIME	REPS

WATER

1L   2L   3L   4L

TODAY'S MOOD

DAILY NUTRITION

Breakfast ________________

Lunch ________________

Dinner ________________

Snacks ________________

TODAY'S MOTIVATION

____

____

● TO START   ✓ OK   → DELAY   ／ STUCK   ✗ CANCEL

NOURISH AND FIT PLANNER

DATE: ___________________________ S M T W T F S

GOALS OF THE DAY

- [ ] _______________________________
- [ ] _______________________________
- [ ] _______________________________
- [ ] _______________________________

WORKHOUT	TIME	REPS

WATER 1L 2L 3L 4L

TODAY'S MOOD

DAILY NUTRITION

Breakfast _______________________
Lunch _______________________
Dinner _______________________
Snacks _______________________

TODAY'S MOTIVATION

____
____

● TO START ✓ OK → DELAY ⁄ STUCK ✗ CANCEL

NOURISH AND FIT PLANNER

DATE: ___________________________ S M T W T F S

GOALS OF THE DAY

- ☐ ....
- ☐ ....
- ☐ ....
- ☐ ....

WORKHOUT	TIME	REPS
☐		
☐		
☐		
☐		
☐		
☐		
☐		
☐		
☐		
☐		
☐		
☐		
☐		
☐		
☐		

WATER

1L 2L 3L 4L

TODAY'S MOOD

DAILY NUTRITION

Breakfast ....

Lunch ....

Dinner ....

Snacks ....

TODAY'S MOTIVATION

....
....

● TO START   ✓ OK   → DELAY   ╱ STUCK   ✕ CANCEL

NOURISH AND FIT PLANNER

DATE: ___________________________ S M T W T F S

GOALS OF THE DAY

- [ ] ___________________________
- [ ] ___________________________
- [ ] ___________________________
- [ ] ___________________________

WORKHOUT	TIME	REPS

WATER

1L 2L 3L 4L

TODAY'S MOOD

DAILY NUTRITION

Breakfast ___________________________

Lunch ___________________________

Dinner ___________________________

Snacks ___________________________

TODAY'S MOTIVATION

____

____

● TO START   ✓ OK   → DELAY   ╱ STUCK   ✕ CANCEL

NOURISH AND FIT PLANNER

DATE: ___________________________   S M T W T F S

GOALS OF THE DAY

- [ ] ______________________________
- [ ] ______________________________
- [ ] ______________________________
- [ ] ______________________________

WORKHOUT	TIME	REPS

WATER

1L   2L   3L   4L

TODAY'S MOOD

DAILY NUTRITION

Breakfast ______________________

Lunch ______________________

Dinner ______________________

Snacks ______________________

TODAY'S MOTIVATION

____

____

● TO START   ✓ OK   → DELAY   ╱ STUCK   ✗ CANCEL

NOURISH AND FIT PLANNER

DATE: ___________________________________ S M T W T F S

GOALS OF THE DAY

- [ ] ___________________________________
- [ ] ___________________________________
- [ ] ___________________________________
- [ ] ___________________________________

WORKHOUT	TIME	REPS

WATER

1L 2L 3L 4L

TODAY'S MOOD

DAILY NUTRITION

Breakfast ___________________________________

Lunch ___________________________________

Dinner ___________________________________

Snacks ___________________________________

TODAY'S MOTIVATION

____

____

● TO START   ✓ OK   → DELAY   ⁄ STUCK   ✗ CANCEL

NOURISH AND FIT PLANNER

DATE: _______________________ S M T W T F S

GOALS OF THE DAY

- ☐ ____________________
- ☐ ____________________
- ☐ ____________________
- ☐ ____________________

WORKHOUT	TIME	REPS

WATER

1L   2L   3L   4L

TODAY'S MOOD

DAILY NUTRITION

Breakfast ____________________

Lunch ____________________

Dinner ____________________

Snacks ____________________

TODAY'S MOTIVATION

____

____

● TO START   ✓ OK   → DELAY   ⁄ STUCK   ✕ CANCEL

NOURISH AND FIT PLANNER

DATE: _______________________________   S M T W T F S

GOALS OF THE DAY

- ☐ _______________________________
- ☐ _______________________________
- ☐ _______________________________
- ☐ _______________________________

WORKHOUT	TIME	REPS
☐		
☐		
☐		
☐		
☐		
☐		
☐		
☐		
☐		
☐		
☐		
☐		
☐		
☐		
☐		

WATER

1L   2L   3L   4L

TODAY'S MOOD

DAILY NUTRITION

Breakfast _______________________________

Lunch _______________________________

Dinner _______________________________

Snacks _______________________________

TODAY'S MOTIVATION

____

____

● TO START   ✓ OK   → DELAY   ／ STUCK   ✗ CANCEL

NOURISH AND FIT PLANNER

DATE: ________________________ S M T W T F S

GOALS OF THE DAY

- [ ] ________________________
- [ ] ________________________
- [ ] ________________________
- [ ] ________________________

WORKHOUT	TIME	REPS

WATER

1L 2L 3L 4L

TODAY'S MOOD

DAILY NUTRITION

Breakfast ________________________

Lunch ________________________

Dinner ________________________

Snacks ________________________

TODAY'S MOTIVATION

____

____

● TO START   ✓ OK   → DELAY   ∕ STUCK   ✕ CANCEL

NOURISH AND FIT PLANNER

DATE: _______________________ S M T W T F S

GOALS OF THE DAY

- [ ]
- [ ]
- [ ]
- [ ]

WORKHOUT	TIME	REPS

WATER

1L 2L 3L 4L

TODAY'S MOOD

DAILY NUTRITION

Breakfast

Lunch

Dinner

Snacks

TODAY'S MOTIVATION

● TO START   ✓ OK   → DELAY   ╱ STUCK   ✕ CANCEL

NOURISH AND FIT PLANNER

DATE: ___________________________   S M T W T F S

GOALS OF THE DAY

- [ ] ___________________________
- [ ] ___________________________
- [ ] ___________________________
- [ ] ___________________________

WORKHOUT	TIME	REPS

WATER

1L 2L 3L 4L

TODAY'S MOOD

DAILY NUTRITION

Breakfast ___________________________

Lunch ___________________________

Dinner ___________________________

Snacks ___________________________

TODAY'S MOTIVATION

____

____

● TO START   ✓ OK   → DELAY   ／ STUCK   ✕ CANCEL

NOURISH AND FIT PLANNER

DATE:

GOALS OF THE DAY

- [ ]
- [ ]
- [ ]
- [ ]

WORKHOUT	TIME	REPS

WATER

1L 2L 3L 4L

TODAY'S MOOD

DAILY NUTRITION

Breakfast

Lunch

Dinner

Snacks

TODAY'S MOTIVATION

● TO START   ✓ OK   → DELAY   ╱ STUCK   ✗ CANCEL